HOPE

April 2017

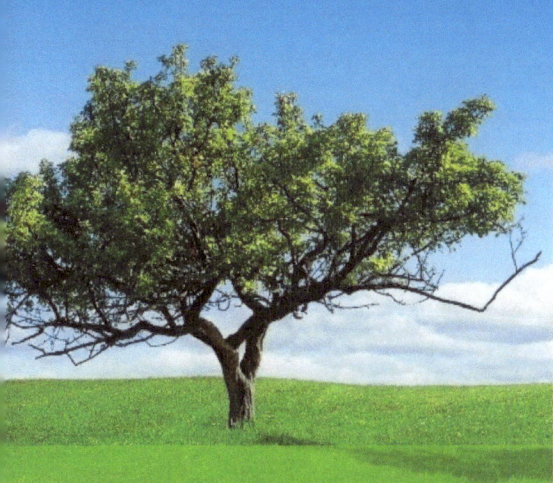

TBI
Advocacy & Education
HOPE
MAGAZINE

"Supporting the Brain Injury Community"

Welcome

TBI HOPE MAGAZINE

Serving All Impacted by Brain Injury

April 2017

Publisher
David A. Grant

Editor
Sarah Grant

Contributing Writers
Ruby Dee
Marci Drimer
Debra Gorman
Scott La Point
Cathy Powers
Charles Ross
Nikki Stang
Shannon Sharman

Amazing Cartoonist
Patrick Brigham

*FREE subscriptions at
www.TBIHopeMagazine.com*

Welcome to the April 2017 issue of TBI HOPE Magazine!

Now in our third year of publication, TBI HOPE Magazine has reached survivors and those who love them, from all over the world. Readers of our publication come from over thirty countries.

Over the years, we have found there to be an unmet need for meaningful information from within the brain injury community. We are grateful to have played a part in meeting that need.

For the first time ever, some of you are holding TBI HOPE Magazine in your hands, reading the print version of our publication.

Last month's soft-launch of TBI HOPE Magazine went off perfectly. We've made a few subtle changes to our format – ensuring easy readership for both our digital as well as our new print readers.

As we move forward, Amazon will remain our distribution partner for the print version. To our loyal digital readers, we will continue to offer TBI HOPE Magazine free of charge to you. Our commitment to serve the brain injury community is stronger than ever.

I always welcome your feedback. Please feel free to email me directly at david@tbihopeandinspiration.com.

Peace,

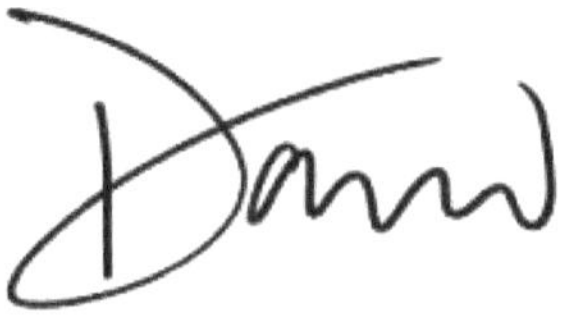

David A. Grant
Publisher

Contents

Supporting the Brain Injury Community Since 2015

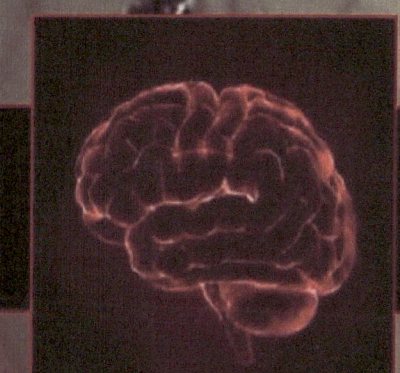

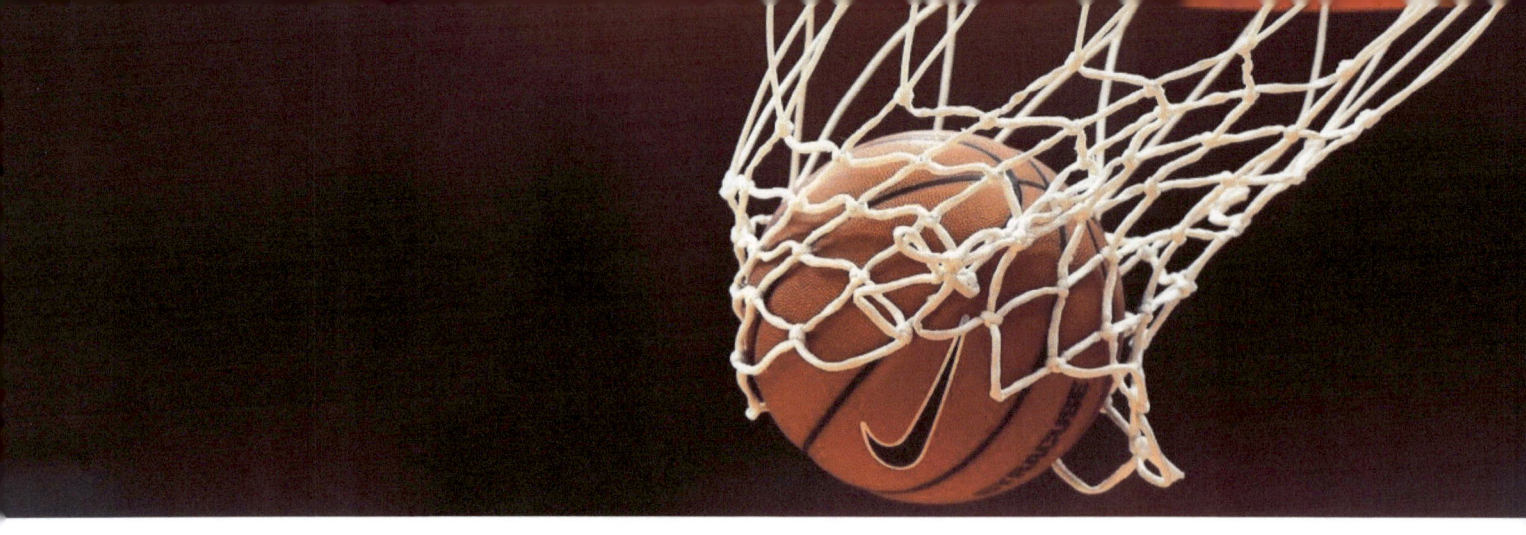

My Basketball Collision

By Nikki Stang

In 2011, I suffered a traumatic brain injury while playing basketball with my P.E. students. A student and I collided while going for the ball and I was head-butted in the mouth. I saw black spots, was dizzy, my hearing was muffled, and my mouth was bleeding substantially. I was worried about losing my front tooth because it took the brunt of the hit and felt loose. The next day I went to the dentist and they said I may have fractured the tooth however, that's hard to see in an x-ray, but if I experienced extreme pain or discoloration in the tooth to let them know.

A month later, when I was on vacation in Las Vegas I noticed my tooth was becoming a murky shade of yellow. When I returned home, I had a root canal to save the tooth. A month later, my tooth was becoming more and more yellow and I was in excruciating pain. When I went back to the dentist, they did another x-ray and saw the tooth fracture, along with a jaw fracture. The dentist ended up pulling my front tooth, and the specialist I saw said I would need an implant and braces. In the meantime, I had frequent migraine headaches, chronic fatigue, and mood swings. I attributed the symptoms to being burnt out from working and attending massage therapy school.

On March 9, 2013, I was admitted to the ICU for 5 days. The night before, my boyfriend and I had gone to a concert and I spent the night at his house. In the morning, I couldn't remember where my clothes were and he said I kept talking but wasn't making any sense. All I wanted to do was lay on the floor. He took me to my parents' house and everyone was asking if I took drugs at the concert; had a date rape drug put in my drink; or suggested maybe I had toxic shock syndrome (TSS).

My parents and boyfriend decided to take me to the hospital because I started losing my balance and strength to stand. I became more and more weak and my head kept dropping forward as my mom was wheeling me in the wheelchair through the hospital. The nurses inserted a catheter to get a urine sample and gave me drugs to calm down because when I was laying in the bed I could not stop squirming around. They performed a CT scan and while we were waiting for the results I started having another episode where I couldn't stop moving my legs and thrashing my head back and forth. At that time, I was taken to the neurology floor. I was put in a bed that had an alarm which would go off if I tried to get up, and the doctors began giving me Keppra, an epileptic seizure drug.

At this point my brother came to the hospital to visit me and I could not recognize him; I thought he was a doctor. My mom was a frantic mess and a nurse pulled her aside and said that my dental history may have something to do with the symptoms I was showing. The doctors felt that they did not have the right equipment or knowledge to test me to see if I had atypical seizures, so I was transported to another neurology department at a different hospital.

To perform the test, nodes on stickers were placed on my head. My family and I found that light and stimulation were triggering my episodes. However, the doctor said that I was not having the correct symptoms to be diagnosed with atypical seizures. The neurologist wanted to give me antipsychotic drugs because he believed these episodes were caused from the sexual abuse I experienced as a child. I refused to believe that my symptoms were caused by that and the neurologist decided it would be best to just discharge me.

At home over the next two weeks I would wake up every morning not knowing who I was. My mom would ask me questions and talk to me for two hours before some memories came back and I was able to remember my life. I had to constantly wear sunglasses because I was so sensitive to light. I was so weak I would get tired from doing simple things like eating or going to the bathroom.

My first Invisalign braces tray arrived and I was reluctant to put them in for a few days but finally decided to try them and wore them overnight. The next morning I woke up knowing who I was for the first time in weeks. My family and I started to realize that the basketball head-butt and mouth injury were related to what was going on with the symptoms I was experiencing with my brain.

My mom made an appointment with an acupuncturist and because of my background with massage, I called my massage school to find a craniosacral therapist. I also began seeing a naturopath, chiropractor, using ionic foot baths, aromatherapy, massage and medical marijuana. My craniosacral therapist recommended I do brain testing because I probably suffered a traumatic brain injury (TBI) from my basketball collision.

> *At home over the next two weeks I would wake up every morning not knowing who I was.*

Meet Nikki Stang

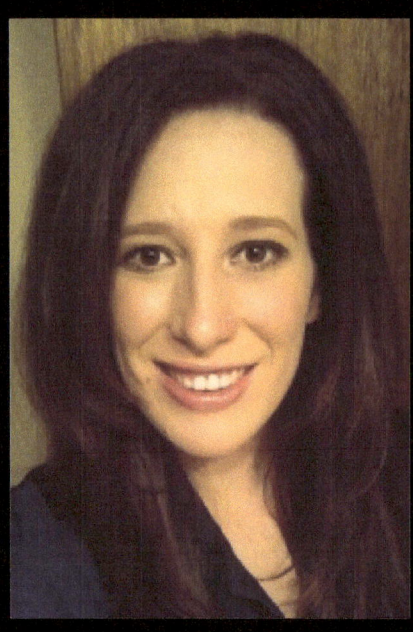

Nikki Stang was born in Denver, Colorado. In 2007 she attended UNLV to start a psychology degree. In fall of 2011 she was accidentally head-butted in the mouth and suffered a traumatic brain injury while playing basketball with her students. Nikki was unaware of her TBI until 2013 when she was later diagnosed shortly after she was pregnant with her first child.

Nikki has recovered from her accident and is now an advocate for brain injury survivors. She has taken classes in aromatherapy and healing touch through ISHA, craniosacral therapy through the Upledger Institute, and heart centered therapy through the Chikly Health Institute.

She is currently living in Denver with her two young children and is a TBI advocate, motivational speaker, and is working on writing a book about her traumatic brain injury experiences.

The neurological psychologist performed 8 hours of brain testing and then diagnosed me with a mild traumatic brain injury.

The diagnosis started my alternative treatment for TBI which became more complicated with the news that I was also pregnant. I would have to go to three appointments a day sometimes to keep myself and the baby stable. I made a promise to myself that once I was stable enough, I would create a website to help others going through the same struggles because there is not much information to help TBI patients.

My website www.mytraumaticbraininjury.com offers information about alternative treatments and provides resources that have helped me in the continuing treatment of my traumatic brain injury.

Things turn out best for the people who make the best of the way things turn out.

~ John Wooden

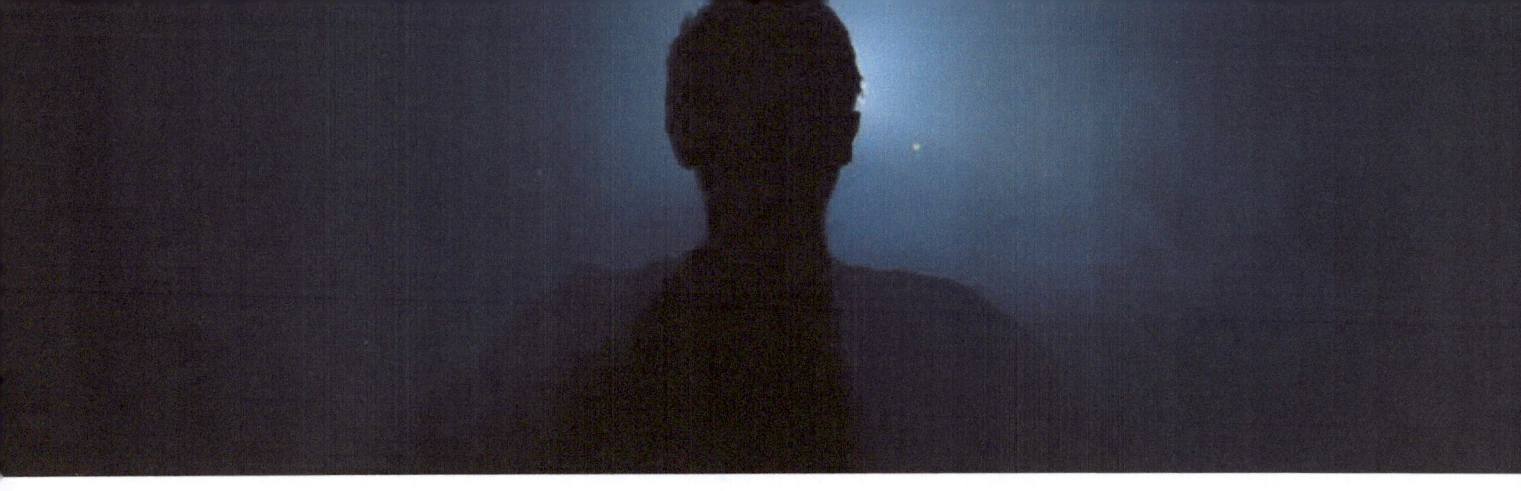

You Can't See Me

By Marci Drimer

You can't see me, but I exist. I live in your neighborhood. I am hurt, and yet you don't seem to know or care. I am broken, and yet you can't see it on my body. I am scared and frightened every day, and yet you will never know. If I told you I had cancer, you would be calling, offering all kinds of help. There would be support groups, survivors with hope, meals delivered, and even child care offered. The phone doesn't ring and the meals don't come.

My eight-year-old daughter cries out, "I want my old Daddy back." "Where did he go?" "Will he ever come back?" She doesn't understand, and can't see his injury. She lives with the effects of his injury every day. It permeates our house and life.

"Sorry Alexa, Daddy can't go swimming, go bowling, ski, run or play."

"Sorry Alexa, Daddy didn't mean to yell at you, he is tired."

"Sorry Alexa, Daddy can't help you with your homework. He is sleeping downstairs."

What are the words I can say to our daughter to explain her old Daddy is gone? There are no words to describe the loss and pain we experience every day.

"I am so tired. Why am I so tired all the time?" I am living with a disease called "Mild" Traumatic Brain Injury, but you can't see it.

My husband and I were hit by a truck while driving our SUV. He was not in a coma and didn't need brain surgery. The MRI looked normal, and he was sent home with the diagnosis of Mild Traumatic Brain Injury. It is invisible to the outside world. If you saw him on the street or had a conversation with him, there would be no visible signs. The only people who know are me, our daughter, and all of his medical care providers. He had ninety-five different therapy appointments within nine months, including vision therapy, speech therapy, physical therapy, psychotherapy, oxygen therapy, vestibular therapy, neuropsychiatric therapy, vocational therapy and on, and on.

There is no end in sight and I am drowning in a brain injury I did not create. It was given to us on a silver platter. We cannot give it back. We are stuck with it for life.

What does all of this mean? I try to find the meaning in the insanity I am living with every day. I sit in Mad Greens typing this story on my computer. People come in and smile at me. They probably think I am doing work. They imagine I work all day and have a family. They don't know that I am living with utter despair and complete brokenness.

This was not the life I imagined when I stood under the chuppah and said, "I do." Where is the white picket fence and husband who kisses me when he returns from a long day at work? Where is the normal life I was supposed to have?

Gone, gone and never coming back. Depression hits me hard and covers me like a heavy blanket. I feel so heavy and defeated. I am powerless. I do not have the inspiration and words of hope to tell myself today.

I ask providers for the name of someone who has been through this nightmare, but no names are given. I called the Brain Injury Alliance and asked for names. The support group organizer has his wife talk to me. "I have a separate life," she tells me. There is a coldness and apathy in her voice. "That will never be me," I tell myself as I hang up the phone. I am alone trying to reach for hope.

This is such a familiar place for me. I am screaming, and yet you can't hear me. God is the only person who brings me comfort during this time. How can I say that? How can a thing, an energy that I can't see, touch or feel bring me comfort? It sounds so cliché, "God is my strength." There is something so beautiful in the peacefulness of surrender. In all of my pain, I see God. In all of my sadness, I feel God. He wraps his arms around me and says, "Don't worry about a thing because everything is going to be alright."

Meet Marci Drimer

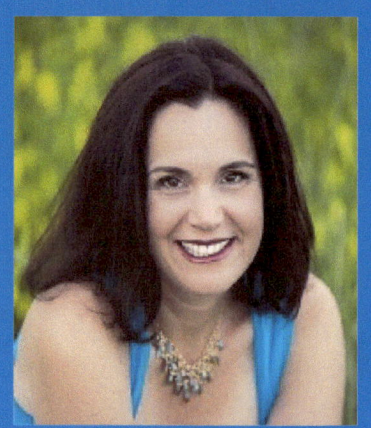

Marci is a Licensed Clinical Social Worker with over 20 years' experience working with anyone who needs to speak their truth. She believes that we can all become experts in creating lives that are happy, joyous and free.

For the past decade she has been a passionate speaker and advocate for survivors of trauma. Marci is also writing a book on this topic entitled "Survivor to Thriver."

"We all have a truth and knowing that lives in our gut. It never lies and always steers you towards your highest good. You have the power to choose the life you want," shares Marci.

We couldn't agree more.

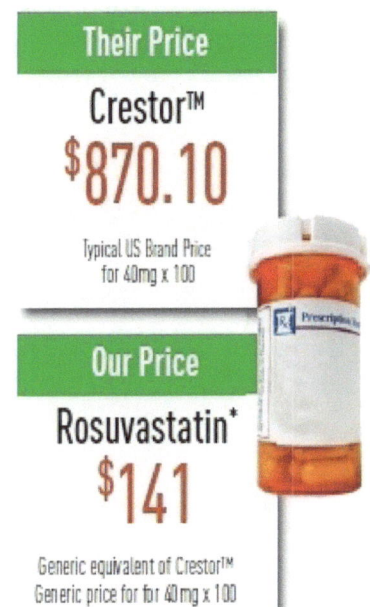
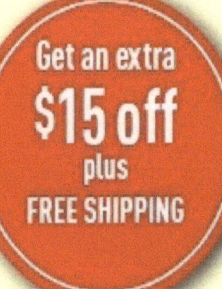
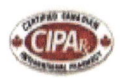 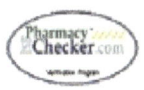 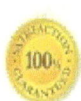 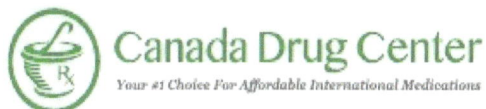

My Story of Inspiration

By Charles Ross

I had my TBI and stroke on November 15, 1985, following a car accident. I was on my way home from a long day of college, during my first semester. I swerved around a truck stopped on the road to make a right-hand turn, on a rainy and very foggy day. I hit a larger car head on, and the truck I swerved around drove off. The woman I hit was not injured, to my knowledge.

An eyewitness came to the car, forced the door open, and held my head up to keep me from choking on my own vomit until the ambulance got there. My mom arrived at the hospital in a nursing uniform; she had come straight from the nursing home where she worked. She had beaten the helicopter there because it had to fly over to Illinois first because of the fog. The hospital staff was talking to the helicopter EMT and she overheard that the paddles were put on me twice. I flew to St. Louis alone, without any other patients, because I was in such dire shape.

After some time in the larger hospital in St. Louis, the doctors told my parents they were removing me from ICU to make room for someone who might live. I was in a coma for fifty days. While in the coma, I drew up into the fetal position and my muscles in my arms and legs shrunk into that position. Initially, I spent more than ten months in the hospital. My first surgery was on my birthday, April 2, 1986. I was in a wheelchair for one-and-a-half years and had seven summers of surgery. Today, I can walk with a cane and I am a left hemiplegic from the stroke.

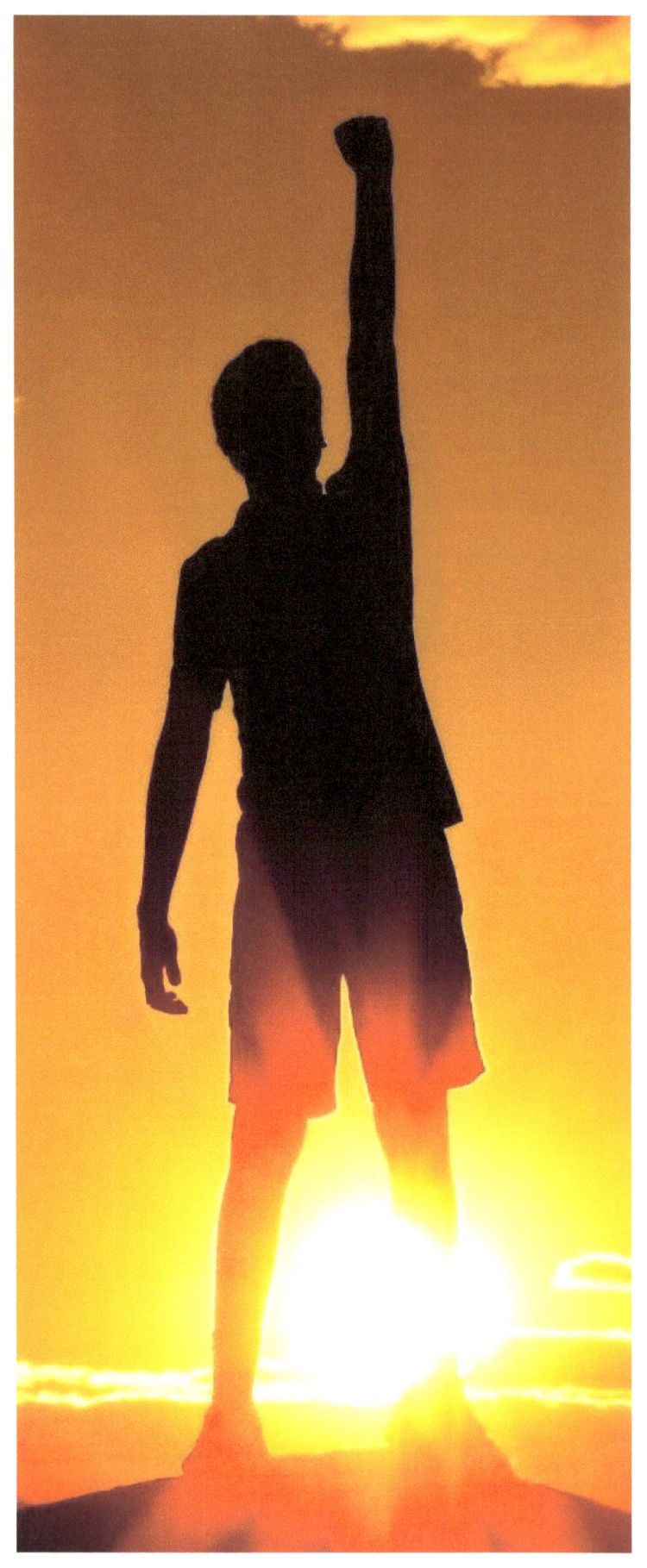

I have severe memory problems. Short term was, and is, still bad today. I had been having what I called "spells", where I would get a feeling like a chill in my spine. My parents took me off seizure medicine because they did not believe I was having seizures. I know those spells increased in frequency after that. I could go days with no spells, but other days I could have hundreds. They would just last a few seconds usually.

As the spells increased, the feelings I had changed too. I began to notice the feeling like I needed to have a bowel movement, though I really didn't. I would get extremely hot, and the sweat would just pour out of me for a few seconds sometimes. Mainly at night, I would wake with the spell and I would have a horrible taste in my mouth. I went to a neurologist and cardiologist and wore monitors at home, but everything was normal, even though I was still having spells.

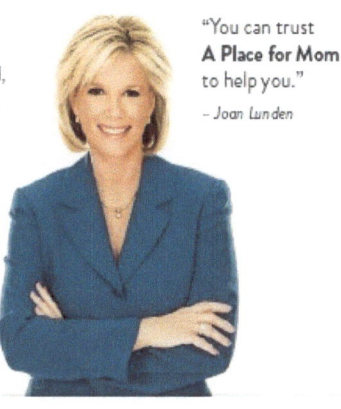
I went back to college after three years. My mom drove and waited on me the first year. When I got my driver's license back, I began driving myself. I was driving to school during the time I still had these spells. I could have been driving, in class, watching TV, walking, sleeping, it did not matter. I never noticed what triggered them. Four years after the accident, in my sleep on New Year's Eve night of 1989, I had a tonic-clonic (grand-mal) seizure. It was determined that those spells were petit-mal seizures. I was diagnosed and treatments began for traumatically-incurred epilepsy.

After I started on medication, the spells decreased dramatically. Each time I had one, my neurologist would increase the medication. Though it helped for some time, the spells never stopped completely. Even though I had the severe memory challenges and physical problems along with the seizures, I managed to get two Associate Degrees over nine years. I was unable to get my Bachelor's degree, with the memory problems.

I started working on my last degree but the stress was too powerful to maintain a job. I began to have "blank" spells. Maybe I had them before, but never remembered or realized it. I realized I had blank spells because while I was driving, I would rear-end someone. I would come out of the blank spell immediately but never remembered what happened, other than the fact that I hit someone. I figured that they hit the brakes quickly in rush hour traffic, and I could not stop.

Over the years, I would have an accident every year or two. Finally, I realized that before each accident I had that strange feeling. After fifteen years of work, I lost my final job. It was so difficult going from job-to-job, learning a new CAD system or way of doing things with my memory problems. I moved in with my parents again. The new neurologist started me on a second medication, which helped. It did not stop the spells though.

I moved again after two years and saw another neurologist who put me on two additional medications. The third medicine was for my spasms and pain, but it was also used to treat seizures. It was not until the fourth medicine was added that the seizures stopped. Altogether, it was over twenty-two years after treatment began and twenty-seven years after the accident, before the right mixture was found and I felt in control again. I moved back in with my parents again, in late 2014.

The medical problems never end for me, it seems. I had back surgery in May of 2016, after going through a trial for a spinal cord stimulator (SCS) in April of 2016, and the trial SCS was successful. My doctor thought a spinal decompression surgery at L4-L5 on the right side would be better than the SCS, as the SCS is a lifetime commitment. That surgery was a failure for my back and right leg pain.

I had my permanent stimulator surgery early in December of 2016. My overall pain has improved, but I am still limited on my standing time and walking distance. These should get better as my strength increases. I was able to do little more than sit on my behind for almost two years, so it will take some time to get my strength back.

I hope my story serves as strength, encouragement, and determination for others with TBI's to never give up. I was never supposed to live! If I did, the doctor's said I would be no more than a vegetable in a chair, unable to do anything for myself.

Today, I am chronicling my story. I drive, I graduated from college with two Associate's degrees, and I worked for fifteen years. There is so much more to the life I've lived since my accident and stroke, but anyone who reads this story should know that anything is possible. You may not accomplish as much as I did, or you may accomplish more. Just know that you should never give up on yourself. Feel proud of what you have accomplished. Never let anyone put shame on you for what has happened to your body. If they were in your shoes, they couldn't do what you can do, and that is SURVIVE! Be proud!

Meet Charles Ross

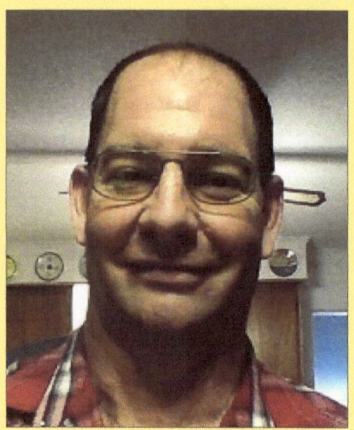

"My name is Charles Ross Jr, and I am a survivor from a brain injury that occurred over thirty-one years ago. I was in a long coma and had to be brought back twice.

I went through many surgeries following the coma to lengthen muscles and tendons in my legs and feet, over several years. They had shortened with damage to the motor control part of my brain. I was in the hospital for almost 11 months initially, but returned for many surgeries.

I spent one-and-a-half years completely in a wheelchair. I now walk with a cane. I also have traumatically induced epilepsy. I wanted to share my entire story, in hopes it could help others going through similar circumstances!"

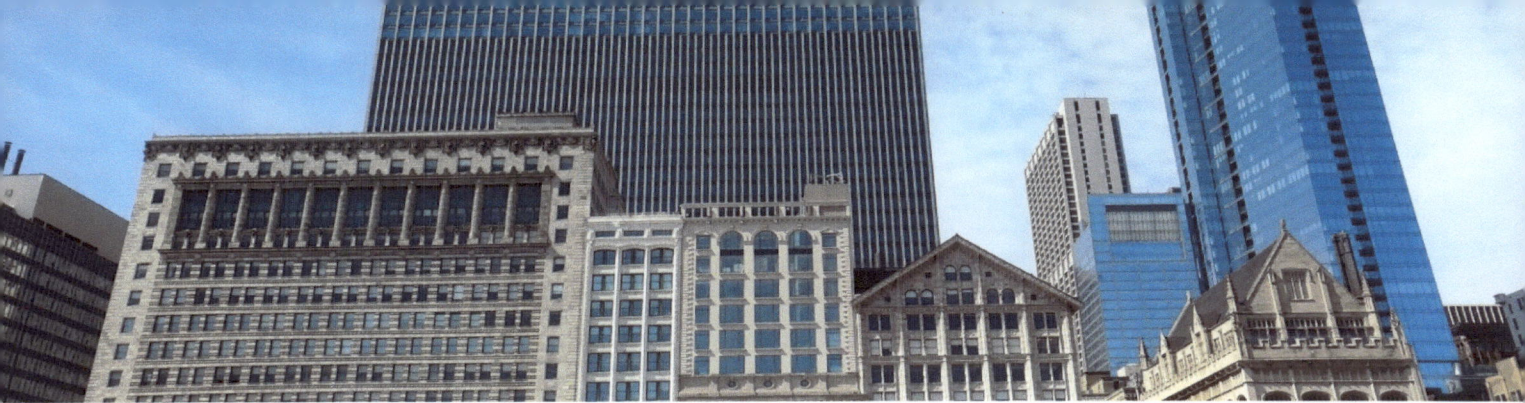

I Miss My Life

By Debra Gorman

I miss my life. That recurring, hurtful thought is one I have had intermittently over the last five years as I navigate my post-brain hemorrhage life. I was fifty-six years old when I died to my old self and began a new journey. Often I do well appreciating what is and being grateful for the opportunity to begin again with new purpose and greater gratitude. Other times, like this afternoon, I get a little too fatigued (common with brain injury) and nostalgia overwhelms me. After all, I spent nearly a lifetime as one person, and now I must make room for someone else to take over; someone with similarities, but many differences and not nearly as capable.

My husband and I relocated to a different part of the country for his work two years ago. Today, I was strolling through parts of downtown with family members. The warm winter sun transported my heart back to my former life with sweet, yet painful, pangs. I remember how different, better, and how "normal" my life was before the cataclysmic event that left me with so many deficits.

As I plodded along on the sidewalks of my new city today, holding onto my husband's arm for stability, I thought about how well I would have known this city by now, prior to my brain injury. Driving was part of my nursing job and I loved being out and about, comfortable driving in any weather, in any traffic. Today, I feel anxiety driving beyond a small area near our home.

There used to be a lilt to my step and I loved walking, long-distance running, backpacking and biking. I had also taken up ballroom dancing and my husband was a graceful partner. Today, I can only walk short distances and my gait feels awkward, unbalanced and I often stagger. I can no longer balance a two-wheeled bicycle.

We entered a gift shop as we strolled through the city. I'm always nervous when I can easily stumble or bump into a rack of breakables. As much as I enjoyed what, for me, was eye candy, I was relieved when we walked out and were not forced to purchase something because of the "you break it, you buy it" rule.

Later, I carefully studied the menu the waitperson handed me in a restaurant. I was not looking for an entree that appealed to me, but rather, closing one eye to read due to double vision, I was searching for something I would not have to cut or have cut for me because I cannot use my dominant hand. Also, I

Meet Debra Gorman

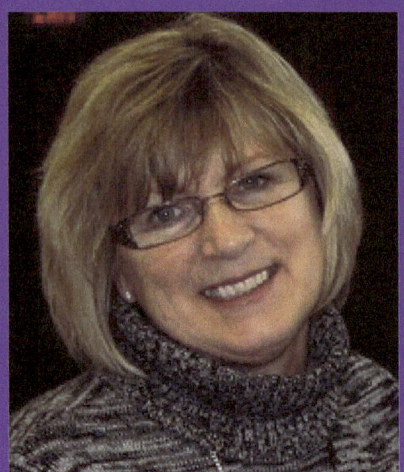

Debra Gorman survived a brain hemorrhage from a brain stem cavernous angioma (a congenital condition), August 2011, at fifty-six years old. She had married the love of her life only six years before her injury.

Three months after the first brain bleed she experienced a subdural hematoma, resulting in a craniotomy. She nearly died several times during those two episodes and family members arrived from all over the country to possibly say goodbye.

Because she survived, she is convinced her life has a new, more focused, purpose. She is grateful to be living, and for the abilities she has retained. She writes a blog entitled Graceful Journey, which she began well before the brain injury, but since then, has focused more on the commonality of suffering.

www.debralynn48.wordpress.com

was looking for something rather spicy because seasoning is all I can taste. How I miss the day when I could order a steak and baked potato, savoring the richness and taking it for granted that I could manage it alone.

Fatigue plays a major role in my life and attitude, but therein lies a dilemma; it is only by pushing oneself that endurance grows. My stamina has certainly improved over the years, but I have only a fraction of my former energy.

I have worked hard to embrace this new chapter of my life and have experienced many blessings and personal growth resulting from dealing with my brain bleed in a positive manner. But I cannot yet say I wouldn't prefer my former life. I hope someday I will feel that way because I will love the person I have become so much more than who I was. Tremendous strides have been made in that direction even if I have an occasional episode, like today, that feels like a setback. Today, there was only enormous sorrow and incredible loneliness. Brain injury affects each person uniquely, so there is no one who can truly understand what I feel or experience.

I try not to beat myself up over what feels like steps backward. My tendency is to be type A: one who wants to get things done promptly and with proficiency. Those traits are not compatible with my new life. Accomplishments now are defined as "some things get done… eventually." Those things will be done to the best of my current ability, which often includes mishaps. I remind myself that it is okay, giving each task my best effort, even if that effort appears sloppy to the casual observer.

My tendency is to compare my injury and emotional progress with others, which is not always helpful. I really want to get this brain injury thing right, whatever right is. Some injured people are so darn cheerful and happy, it irks me. I want someone to express how difficult this life is and how much it hurts. That would make me feel better, to know I'm not alone in my struggle. For some reason, that type of real-ness encourages me to keep striving forward and practicing the discipline of gratitude.

I plan to go to bed early tonight and wake up refreshed tomorrow, ready to face a new day, a day closer to loving my new life.

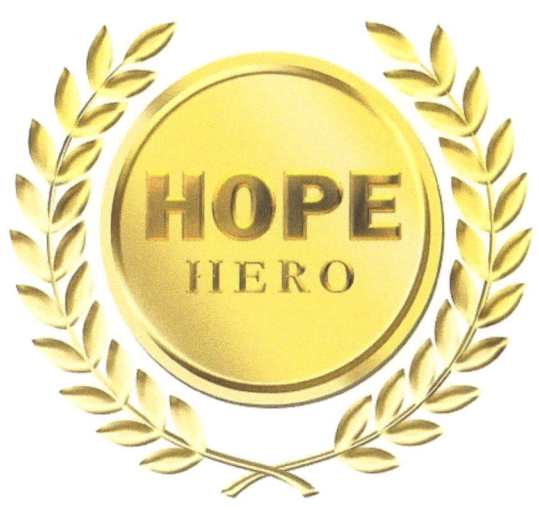

Introducing The Hope Hero Award

Every month, the TBI HOPE Network will recognize an individual from within the brain injury community with the HOPE HERO Award. The recipient of the award will be recognized for selfless service in the brain injury community.

Who can qualify?

Anyone with a direct connection to brain injury. Recipients need not be familiar names. Know of a survivor who is making a difference in the lives of others? How about a caregiver or family member who has gone above and beyond? Anyone can qualify as a Hero nominee.

How do I Nominate a Hero?

Send an email to myhero@tbihopeandinspiration.com. In 300 words or less, describe your Hero and why you think he/she should be recognized. Be sure to include a photo of your Hero as well.

How do I Know if my Hero has been recognized as a HOPE HERO?

The monthly award recipient will be featured in TBI HOPE Magazine. We'll include a photo as well as details about why they were selected. We will also announce the recipient on our Facebook page. Recipients will also receive a digital Certificate of Appreciation by email suitable for printing and framing.

No one recovers from a brain injury alone. Here's your opportunity to let others know about your Hero!

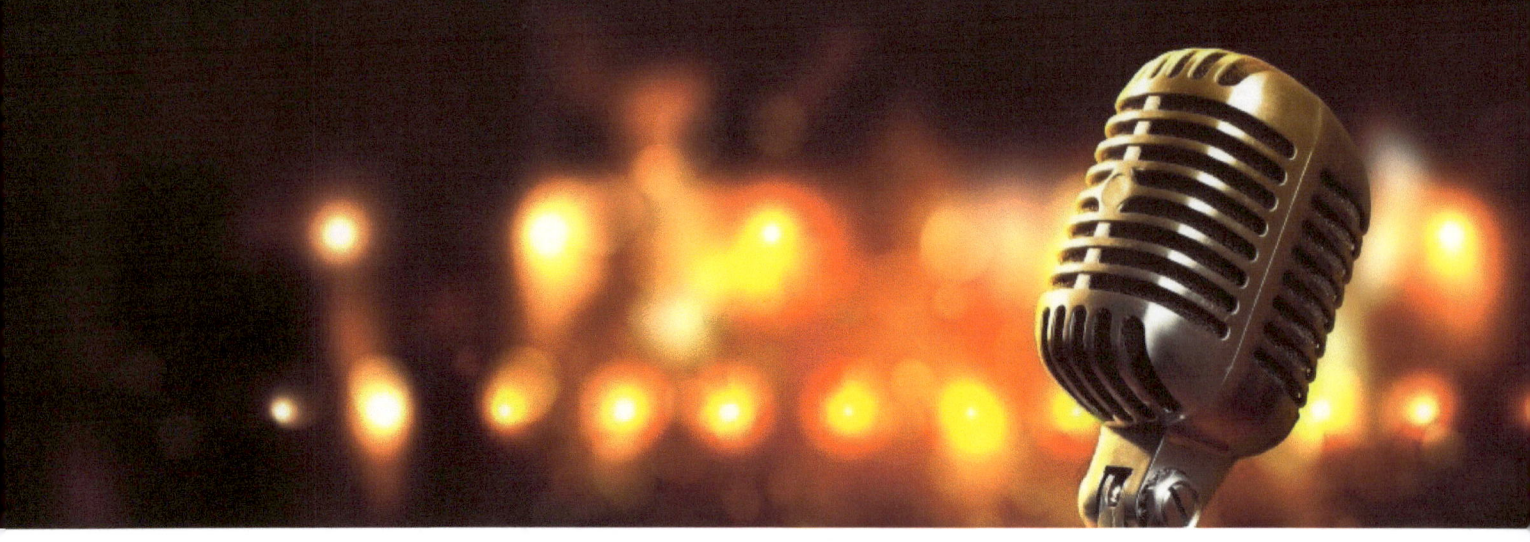

What am I Singing?

By Ruby Dee

I am a traumatic brain injury survivor. I'm not a wounded warrior or athlete, just a gal who was riding my scooter at the wrong place at the right time. And eight years later, I'm finally able to write about it. That is, I'm finally able to again access the side of my brain that deals with language, and am able to find most of my vocabulary- after a long, difficult and dark recovery when that side of my brain seemed lost to me forever.

Eight years ago, I was driving down the road, when the driver of a car didn't see me and pulled into the street. I made the appropriate evasive maneuver, but my front tire hit a pothole, and I went head over heels, landing on my head. Even with a full helmet, the impact was severe enough that I was knocked unconscious. Luckily, the driver behind me was a doctor and she pulled over, called 911, covered me with a blanket, and made sure I wasn't choking on my own blood (I'd bitten through my tongue).

I was lucky. I woke up in the emergency room eight hours later, confused and rambling, but alive. I went home, and there the ordeal began. After a head injury like this, you can feel almost fine right away. But then as the days go by, symptoms start to creep in, making you more and more 'brain-injured'. At first, I felt like I had a bad headache, and was nauseous. Then, I began to feel extreme vertigo- I needed to touch the wall or a chair or something to make sure I didn't go crashing to the floor any time I tried to walk to the bathroom or kitchen. And then my brain seemed to unravel from there.

I became extremely confused and easily distracted. All noises seemed to just babble at me- whether that was the TV or my husband talking to me. I couldn't easily understand what was being said to me. And the written word became a jumble. I love to read and had figured since I wasn't very mobile, I could at least get some reading in. But no. When I looked at the printed page, all the words fractured and moved around- my eyes couldn't settle on any string of words that made sense, no matter how hard I concentrated. So watching movies or reading anything were both out.

And then I began to forget words. Not actually forget them- more like just not able to access them. I could see the picture of the thing I wanted to say- a friend's face or an image of a table, for example. But I just couldn't find the word. I knew that I knew the word, but it just wasn't there. Most words weren't there. So writing, let alone speaking clearly, were both out too.

I'm a songwriter. My band, Ruby Dee and the Snakehandlers actually had a series of shows for our CD release the weekend after my accident. Since I couldn't talk to any specialists right away, I called my regular doctor. She told me that I should perform those shows if at all possible, as music somehow helps the healing process for all types of brain injuries. They don't know why, but for some reason, the rhythm and cadence and musical-language-muscle memory helps the brain lift weights and recuperate.

So, I performed. I needed help up onto the stage and had to hold on to a barstool so I wouldn't fall over. Throughout each song, I would suddenly stall in the middle of a line and completely forget what I was singing. I started bringing my lyric sheets on stage to avoid complete lyrical failure.

> "Throughout each song, I would suddenly stall in the middle of a line and completely forget what I was singing."

I don't remember that window of time. There are 'photographs' in my mind of something I did or a friend's face, but for the better part of two years, I don't recall conversations, things I did, people I saw- no details at all. During that time, I went to neurologists, neuropsychologists, and other brain doctors. I took tests. I was told to take it easy and give it time. But they couldn't tell me how much I would get back if any, of my brain at all.

I've always been someone who felt that who I was in the world was reflected less by my looks and more by my intelligence. Suddenly, I couldn't access a good part of my cognitive function- I couldn't communicate clearly, couldn't read nor write easily, and became so confused and forgetful that I felt like I really wasn't here anymore. Or I might as well not be.

I became severely depressed and even contemplated suicide a few times. For, on top of the weight of not being who I'd always identified myself as being- an intelligent, communicative person- I received almost no support for the injury and all its side effects. After the initial doctor's visits, I was told there was nothing they could do. No one suggested cognitive therapy. No one suggested anything.

Years passed like this. I spent a lot of time in bed, depressed, weeping, not knowing what, if anything, I could do. I couldn't wait tables, as I couldn't remember what people had ordered, or who'd ordered what. I couldn't manage an office, or work in a store where there were lots of noises and movement. I became distracted and confused and fatigued so easily, I couldn't really do much. Then two things happened that started to turn my life around. I got the insurance company to agree to send me to a cognitive therapist. Even with the intense difficulty I experienced reading, I did a LOT of research online about head injuries, and read that cognitive therapy seemed to help in many cases. It would take me days to read through an article, but I plowed ahead and persevered. The insurance company sent me to one cognitive therapy appointment. Then they told me they didn't see any results so they denied any further appointments. After one session.

But that one session helped. A lot. The doctor had given me word games and exercises to do, and even after being cut off from returning to see her again, I realized that I could find other word games and exercises on my own.

Sure, I couldn't speak or write like I used to be able to. And my efforts to get help had been shot down, and no suggestions or advice had been given to me for outreach or support of any kind, so I felt completely alone. And I still became easily confused, fatigued, and distracted. And words, for the most part, still eluded me. But if I pushed myself hard, I could do little things like research online, no matter how long it took me to get it done. And I could work hard at word games and exercises I found online, and on apps on my phone. So bit by bit, truly inch by inch, I began to climb out of the depression, and start to fight my way back to better cognitive function.

Before the accident, songs would just come to me- lyrics, music and all. Maybe just a snippet of a tune, or a phrase from a film or something someone said or that I read somewhere. But pretty quickly, I would feel the rhythm of the words tell me what the music should sound like, or the music would inform me of the lyrics. Either way, songs came pretty quickly and effortlessly.

After the accident, after years of doing word games and exercises, writing stories and recipes and radio shows, one day a few lyrics with a tune came into my head, and it floored me. It had been so long since that had happened that I immediately dropped what I was doing and wrote out those few lyrics, and then

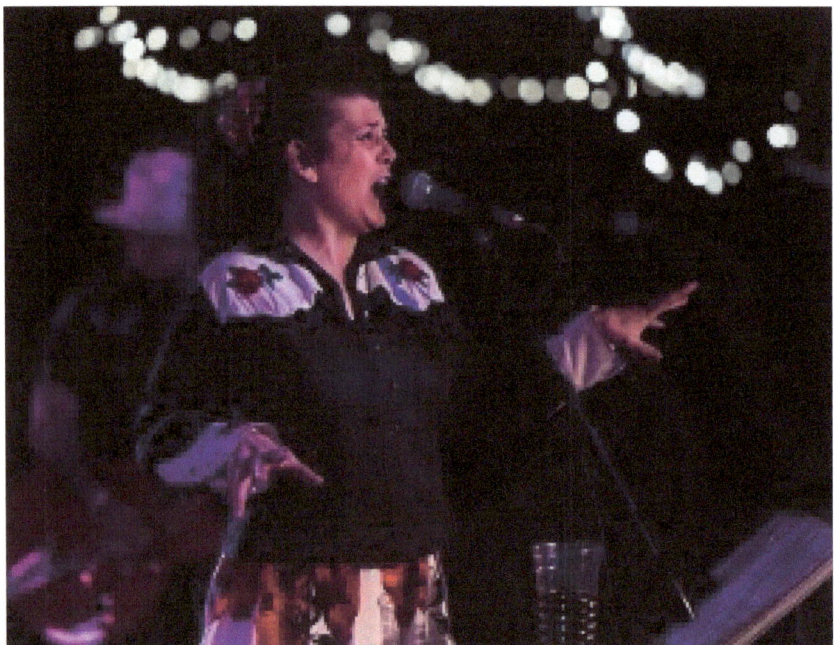

pushed myself to work at it until the song began to take shape.

And suddenly I was writing songs again. Not easily, and not effortlessly. I really have to work at a song now. I might have a snatch of tune or a line or two that sounds like something going around and around in my head, so I write that down, then let it percolate. I come back to it and work out the song: what is the song trying to say? What is the story? What is the feel? Is it happy, or sad, or angry? What is the final message I want to get across?

Best of all are the connections I've made with numerous folks across the globe- people who have either experienced a head injury personally or have a friend or family member with some sort of TBI. I'm able to pass along all the information I've gleaned over the past eight years- contacts, articles, groups that help folks with head injuries, even a Facebook group for those suffering from TBI.

Anything I can do to help ease someone else's journey down this long, dark, painful road makes me feel just a bit better about having to go it nearly alone. If I can help someone else avoid all that self-doubt and suffering and let them know that yes it's hard right now, but trust me, it will get easier in time, then great. I'm ok with having gone through it too.

I still get tired easily, and I'm very distracted and confused in noisy, bustling places. I can perform at shows but can't easily hang out before or after. The music and voices and movement wear me down to a nub. I still need my lyric sheets in front of me. I can get through most of a song without the crutch, but then suddenly find myself in the middle of a song and think "What am I singing?" I can speak much more clearly now and am able to read and write with a lot more ease (yay!). Sure, songs take longer to write- even writing this article took all of a day. But the fact that I can write again, that I can communicate my thoughts and feelings, that's all a gift for which I will never stop being grateful.

I can't do all of what I used to be able to do, but what I can still do, I'm going to do really well, and for as long as I'm able.

The greatest discovery of all time is that a person can change his future by merely changing his attitude.

~ *Oprah Winfrey*

Meet Ruby Dee

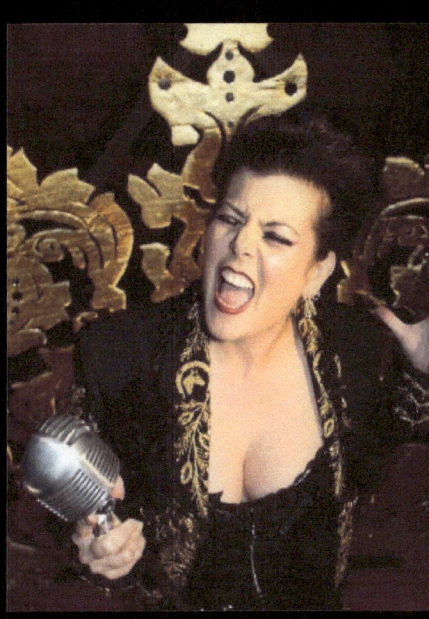

Ruby grew up in the foothills of Northern CA and the panhandle of Texas, riding horses in the back woods near Folsom Prison, and singing with family on the back porch. She attended university at fifteen, helped found the North Coast California Earth First! and fished professionally in Alaska. Eventually, Ruby moved to Seattle, WA where she opened a series of restaurants. She transitioned from restaurateur to singer/songwriter when she started Ruby Dee and the Snakehandlers in 2002.

Thrice Grammy-considered, Ruby Dee and the Snakehandlers tour the world, and produce award-winning records, despite the fact that Ruby suffered a moderately severe brain trauma several years ago that left her unable to complete sentences, let alone write. She fought her way back from that accident, and is now able to communicate and write award-winning songs again.

Ruby continues to write and sing to her heart's content.

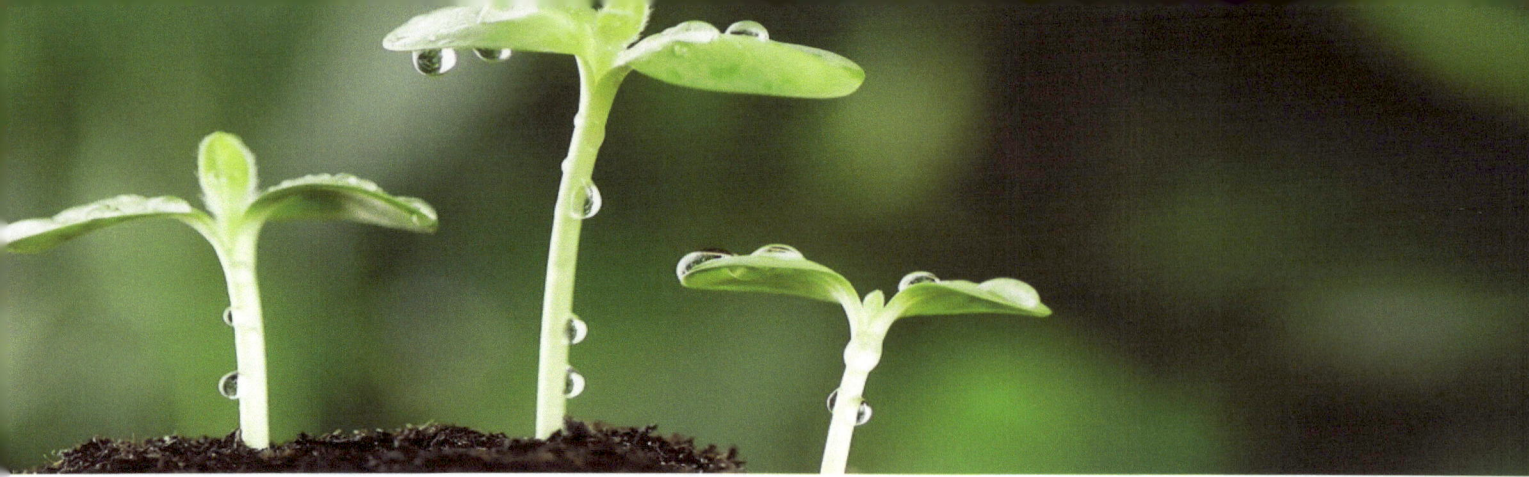

Nurture the Living

By Cathy Powers

What if you had two fruit trees and one of them died? Would you continue to nurture them both? You had personally devoted many years loving, caring for, and shaping these amazing fruit trees! You looked forward to watching both trees produce beautiful fruit for many years. But, one tree has died. Would this change your plans for the future?

When the first tree died unexpectedly, would you find a way to accept your painful loss and then give 100% of your time and resources to the tree left living? Or, would you insist on spending the rest of your days giving half (50%) of your time and resources to each, the living and the dead tree? I think we can all agree it would be foolish to continue taking care of the dead tree. So, let's take it to a deeper level.

What if one of your two children died? Would you continue to nurture them both? Why is it that when a loved one passes away, it's so hard for you and I to accept the loss? Why do we struggle to let them go? Once a person dies, is there anything we can do to bring our loved one back? The answer is no. So, if we are capable of realizing that taking care of a dead tree is pointless, why do we not arrive at the same conclusion about a loved member of the family who has died?

Since the beginning of time, we are all appointed a day and hour to pass from this life. Not one of us can escape death. Yet when death comes, and especially when it is unexpected and our loved one seemed to have many years left to live, many of us insist on carrying the dead around with us for the rest of our lives, showing them off to anyone who will let us, and not focusing on the loved ones still living. Our living loved ones deserve our time and attention.

As a grieving mother who has lost a precious adult child far too early, I now share that I wish I'd had the capacity to see this truth earlier—that our living loved ones need, deserve, and want our time and attention—as clearly as I see it now. I wish I could go back and give my daughter 100% of my "Momma heart" instead of the 50% I gave her, thinking that the other 50% of my time and attention still belonged to her big brother no longer living.

It's been quite a challenge for me to learn how to better balance my grief journey, staying present and continuing to walk forward in this life without my son. I am blessed to have a wonderful husband and loving daughter, who both deserve to have me whole and as healthy as possible on a daily basis. Taking time to honor and remember our loved ones is healthy.

Just because my son, who was serving his country, has passed away from this world does not mean that I should move on, forget him, or quit sharing my wonderful memories of his life. My memories of him will always be with me, and I believe it's healthy to share his life stories, in moderation, with others willing to listen. As long as I live, I will set aside special time to honor and remember him, and I will continue to love him always, knowing I will one day see his beautiful smiling face again. This, more than anything else, brings me great joy and peace. What is one of the things you are willing to do for the living around you?

Sowing into people's lives can be as simple as a smile, being a good listener, donating something you no longer use, or want to keep, to a charity. Or, be kind to someone expecting nothing in return. What are you willing to do for the living around you?

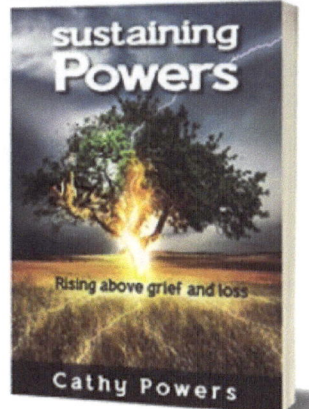

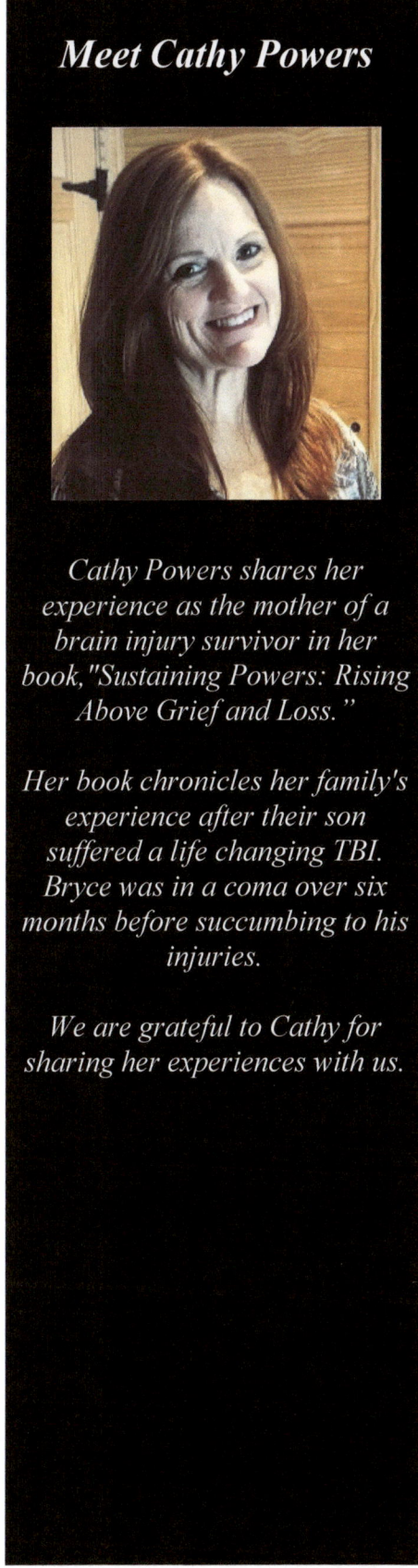

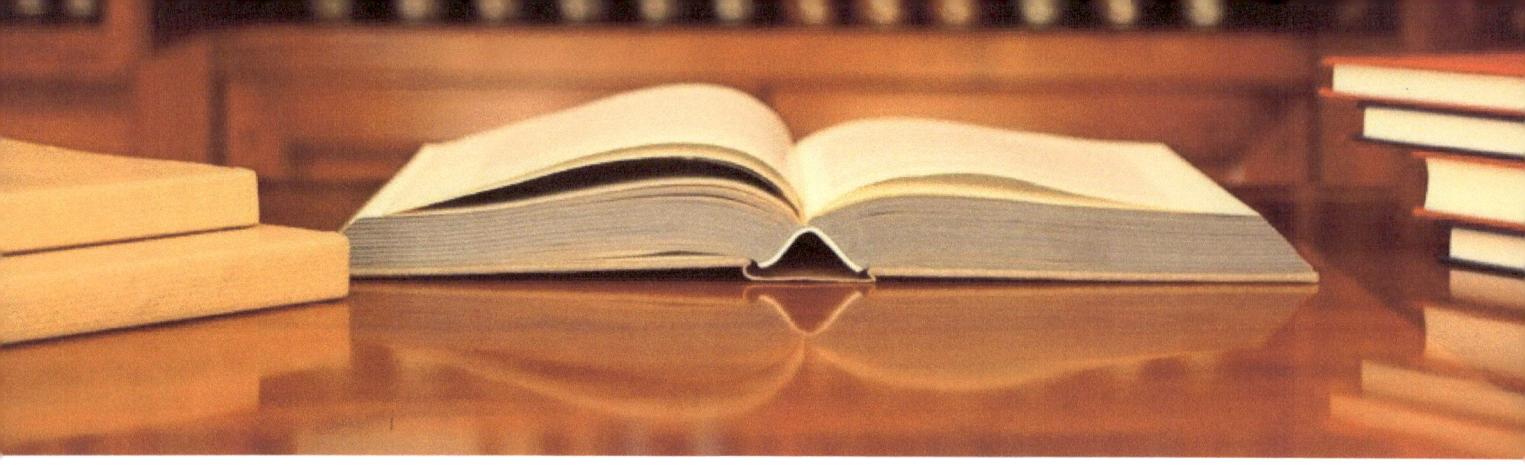

Further Learning

By Shannon Sharman

I am the happiest I have ever been. Who would have known? It took so long to get over the depression of having lost my old life. I actually never thought I would get over it. However, I don't worry about the small things anymore. I try to remind myself to see the people I want to see more, as they are not there forever and it has made for happier times.

I did not get into a Paramedics course at University as planned. It turns out my Diplopia (double vision) was too bad to make the cut. I applied in 2016 for an Enrolled Nursing course. I successfully got in! I have loved it. I have learned so much through the course. I train at the hospital where I work so I can work/study all in the same place. I have already completed six months and two placements. I will be graduating as an Enrolled Nurse in December 2017. My intention is to work in Emergency at the hospital which saved my life. However, there are so many possibilities for a future career in Nursing.

I was wearing an eye patch for my double vision full time however, I was getting picked on every day. It caused me to feel bad about myself. After much brainstorming with my Optometrist, we decided to trial different contact lenses in my eyes so that I could work without an eye patch. I still have to wear it when I drive as I worked hard to get my license back six months ago. There is no freedom like being able to drive whenever you like. I am so happy I can choose to drive rather than get the bus everywhere. My gait is unsteady and when I catch the bus (as I don't have a visible disability), I am not offered a seat from other passengers. This can become frustrating, especially when I am asked to move to accommodate other passengers. It is just easier to drive places!

I did get married in December 2015. It was the best day of my life. Some of my family came from different parts of Australia to be there, including my Grandparents from Western Australia. I could not include all my amazing friends, but I thought of them, as I had so much support during my sickness, from them. We just did not have the money to have a huge gathering. It was very good though and a happy day.

I do have many symptoms I live with daily from my Brainstem Cavernoma (which I named Timmy) and the shunt I, unfortunately, have in my head. However, this is part of life that reminds me how much I have been through. It has been an absolute pleasure to get comments from people that I don't look like I have a brain injury. I feel I struggle with words as the day goes on and I really notice it, but it's nice others don't see this.

I have worked so hard over the past six months to complete a whole semester of study. It was hard and it took all my strength and many painkillers to get through the first six months. I will keep going as I want to reach graduation.

I am happy and I cannot imagine having had a life without brain injury. I thoroughly enjoy meeting new people who have been through a similar journey as me and can talk for hours about brain injury. The only downfall is that Queensland had a fabulous campaign in our brain injury awareness month (August), called BangonaBeanie. This was amazing and I looked forward to it every year, but it was cancelled last year.

The only advice I have to Australian TBI sufferers (especially Queenslanders), Google STEPS. They are a support group for brain injury survivors and they are amazing. My life wouldn't be the same without them.

I have had so many milestones and things I was told I couldn't do: I started walking again, I started working again, and I started studying again. I got married; I was chief bridesmaid at my best friend's wedding. The biggest thing is that I am allowed to drive again. Anything is possible! I've also participated in many charity walks and events. Life is good.

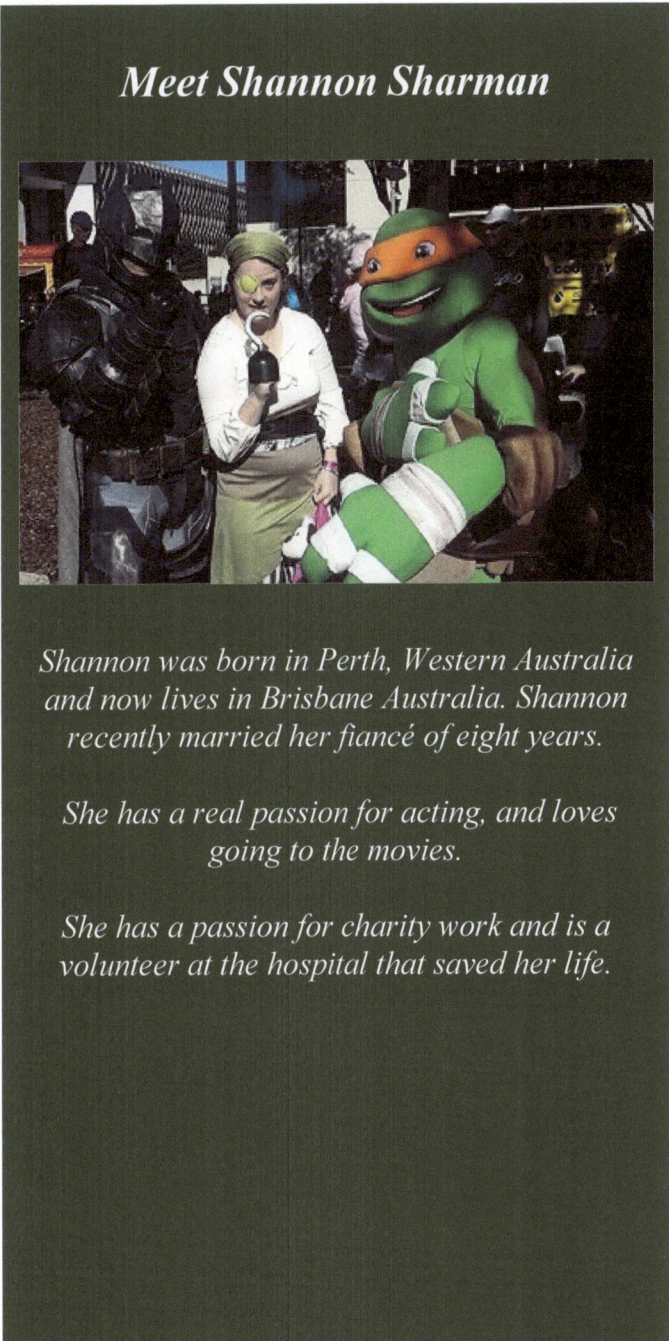

Meet Shannon Sharman

Shannon was born in Perth, Western Australia and now lives in Brisbane Australia. Shannon recently married her fiancé of eight years.

She has a real passion for acting, and loves going to the movies.

She has a passion for charity work and is a volunteer at the hospital that saved her life.

Attitude is a little thing that makes a big difference.
-Winston Churchill

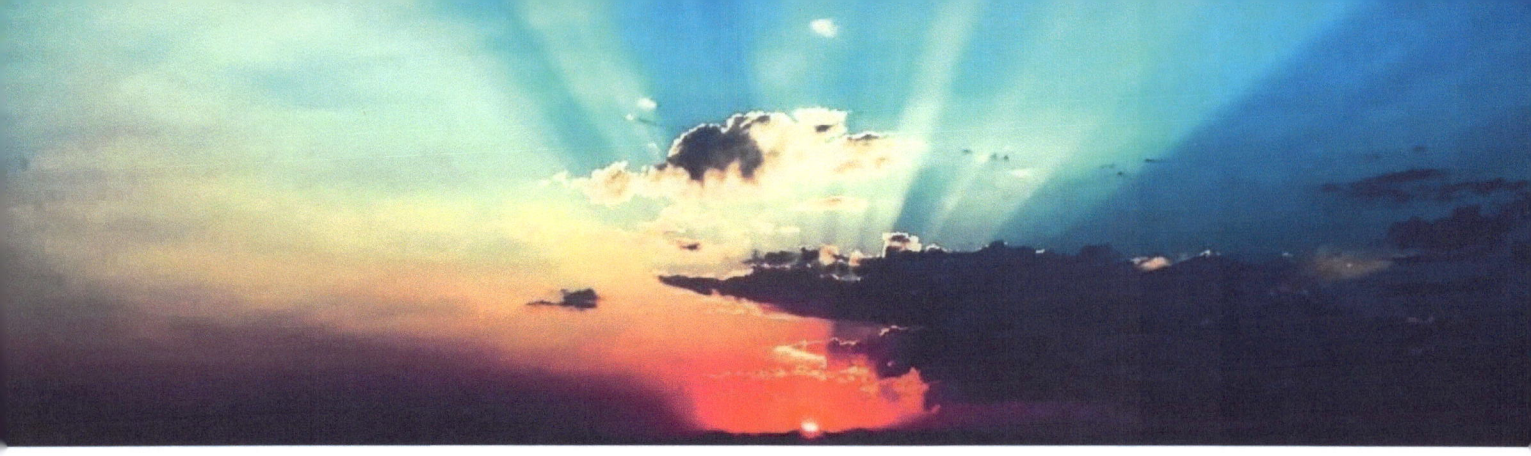

It's Who You Are, Not What You Do
By Dr. Scott La Point

It's who you are, not what you do, that gives life meaning. For every load of laundry he folds and carpet he vacuums, for every day spent cleaning and mopping and scrubbing, the nagging question remains: Who am I?

This isn't how he planned to live out his days post-injury, emptying the dishwasher every morning and tidying up bedrooms and bathrooms. But Jonathon* isn't alone. For most, if not all, of the members of a support group in Northern Colorado, the question of "Who am I now that I have a brain injury," gets harder and harder to answer as income dwindles and influence disappears and sleep worsens; as doubts about worth and significance and importance hang around longer than expected. Dreams of shaping the future of aerospace or returning to a career as a school nurse or designing pages for a daily newspaper come plummeting to earth as reality takes hold; as damaged neurons and deficits in executive functioning, processing speed and memory, as well as changes in personality alter the person's sense of who he or she is.

But that isn't how it should – or needs – to be. As seven individuals with brain injury and three care partners/caregivers discussed at the support group's twice-monthly meeting, the idea that who someone is, post-TBI/ABI, has less to do with vocation and ability and aptitude than it does with purpose and meaning, with "Why am I here," and "Why does my life matter?"

The proposition that someone's life can be as meaningful and vital and remarkable after brain injury, regardless of what he or she does – or doesn't do – was one proposed by a member who told the group that a person's worldview determines how he or she views all of life and reality – and disability. "We all have a set of values and beliefs around which we organize our lives," said the member, who works as a psychologist, but identified himself as a person and a husband and a father. Oh, and he survived a severe TBI more than 20 years ago – along with seven years of graduate school.

"Our culture tries to tell us that unless we're producing or unless we're doing something constructive or meaningful, our lives don't have value and we don't matter. But I want to challenge you," he said to those in attendance. "Your life has value, period. Whether you're folding socks or building rockets, nursing kids at school or still wondering what to do as someone with a brain injury, your life matters. You matter. Unfortunately, we as a society have forgotten that we're human beings, not human doings."

For Jonathon, he still vacillates between wanting what was and accepting what is, and that's okay. In time he'll make a decision that's in line with his worldview and his unshakable faith in God. For another member, falling 40 feet and bouncing off the cement at the age of 17 altered his life's trajectory, but it didn't destroy his identity or his faith in God or in himself.

While Anthony* still struggles with anger and with diminished self-worth, and he forgets more than he remembers, one thing he hasn't forgotten is that God has a purpose and a plan for his life. In fact, beginning in two weeks, Anthony and his wife will be facilitating a group at a church in Loveland for individuals who have a disability, their family, and other interested parties. He has discovered that despite his disability, he matters, and his life still has value.

So, whether you're home folding socks and underwear all day or working part-time delivering packages for FedEx or trying to re-write your life as you continue to struggle with fatigue and dizziness and a shattered sense of self, our group exists so that you can learn to live as someone who has survived a brain injury and everything else life throws at you, with your identity intact, because remember, what you do for a living doesn't matter. It's who you are that does!

Names have been changed to protect the person's identity.

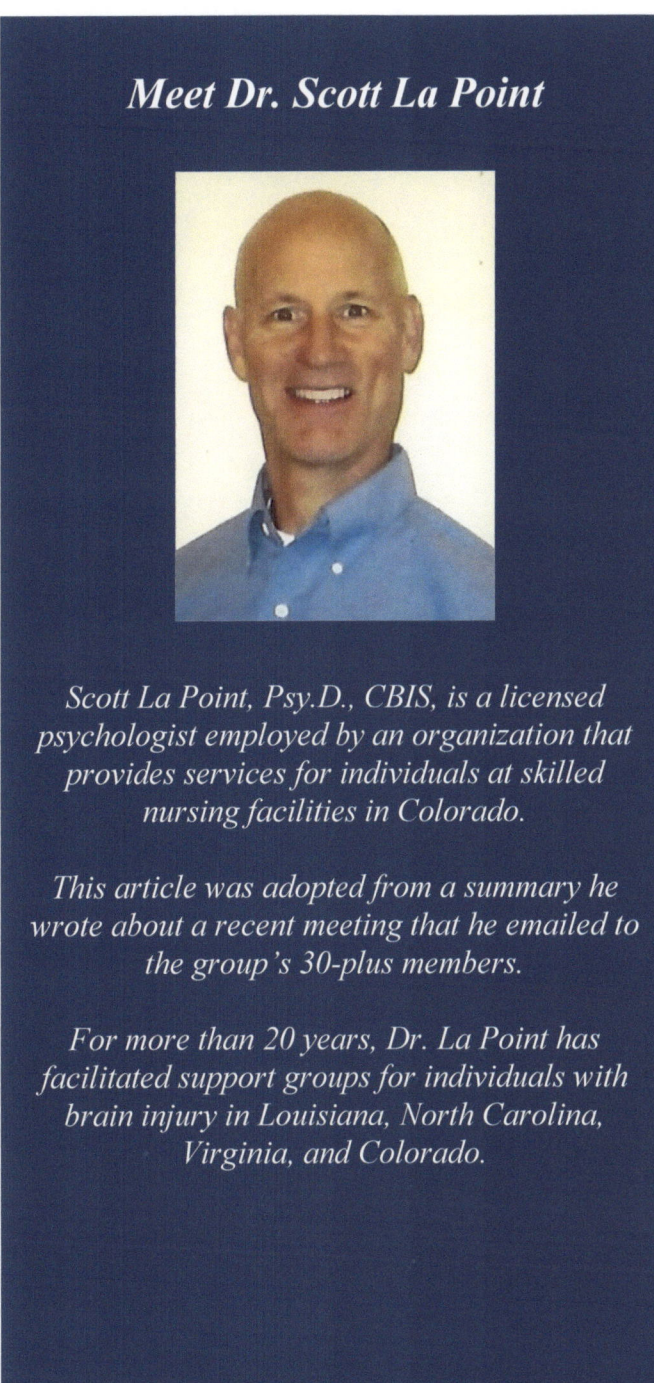

Meet Dr. Scott La Point

Scott La Point, Psy.D., CBIS, is a licensed psychologist employed by an organization that provides services for individuals at skilled nursing facilities in Colorado.

This article was adopted from a summary he wrote about a recent meeting that he emailed to the group's 30-plus members.

For more than 20 years, Dr. La Point has facilitated support groups for individuals with brain injury in Louisiana, North Carolina, Virginia, and Colorado.